MIND STRONG, BODY STRONG

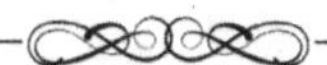

A Science-Backed Blueprint for Energy, Clarity, and Thriving in Midlife and Beyond

Dr. Paulette Lewis, DPT

Doctor of Neurological Physical Therapy

Health & Wellness Coach | Consultant | Educator

COPYRIGHT

© 2026 by Paulette Lewis.

Publisher: Paulette Lewis, DPT

Publisher website: www.paulettelewisdpt.com

Author website: www.paulettelewisdpt.com

Printed in the United States of America

ISBN: 979-8-9961156-0-0

First edition: 2026

Medical disclaimer: "This book is intended for informational purposes only and does not constitute medical advice. Readers should consult a qualified healthcare provider before beginning any exercise, nutrition, or wellness programs.

ACKNOWLEDGEMENTS

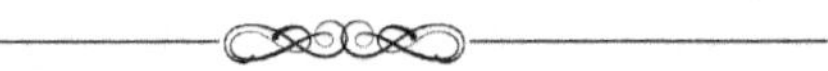

There is a saying I have heard many times throughout my life, and one that I have come to know as an absolute truth: it takes a village. Writing this book confirmed that for me in ways I did not fully anticipate when I sat down to begin it. No page of Mind Strong, Body Strong exists in isolation — every word has been shaped by people who loved me, challenged me, supported me, or trusted me with their care. This is my attempt to honor them.

First and foremost, I give all glory and honor to God. I am a woman of faith, and that faith has been the floor I have stood on in every difficult season — including the seasons during which this book was written. When motivation was low, faith carried me. When I doubted whether my story was worth telling, faith reminded me that it was not my story alone to keep. I am grateful beyond measure for the grace that has guided every step of this journey.

To my husband Lee— my partner, my teammate, my person through more than two decades of life together. You have never once made me feel that my ambitions were too large or my dreams unrealistic. Even in our most difficult seasons — and we have had them — you have been steady. You have given me the space to be a clinician, a coach, a speaker, a business owner, and now an author, while also being your wife and the mother of our children. I do not take that lightly. Not for a single day. Thank you for every sacrifice, seen and unseen.

To my daughter and my son, Loren and Philip — you are my greatest motivation and my most honest mirrors. Watching you both navigate your own journeys — your college years, your high school halls, your growing independence — has reminded me over and over again why it matters to model what it looks like to pursue your best life without excuses and without apology. I hope this book shows you what is possible when you commit to your purpose, even when life makes it inconvenient. I love you both more than words can hold.

To my parents, John and Elfreda — thank you for giving me the foundation that made everything else possible. The values instilled in me growing up, the discipline, the love of learning, and the knowledge that excellence is always worth the effort — all of it lives in these pages. To my maternal grandmother, whose words I carry with me every day: you were right. When you have health and strength, you truly are rich. I write in your honor.

To Dr. Katrina Banks, DPT — my colleague, my collaborator, my friend. Our Neurowellness Conversations podcast has been one of the great joys of this chapter of my career. You challenge me intellectually, you support me personally, and you remind me consistently that the work we do together extends far beyond the clinical walls we each operate within. Thank you for your expertise, your authenticity, and your unwavering belief in rest as power — a message this world desperately needs. I am grateful to do this work alongside you.

To Dr. Gathline Etienne, MD – my colleague and friend. You showed me respect and resilience and made me feel as though I could conquer anything I put my mind to. You push me to be the best in all I do, and you support me immensely. I thank you for it.

To my clinic staff — thank you for showing up, for caring for our patients with the same dedication I try to model, and for holding things together on the days when the weight of building something meaningful felt heavier than usual. You are not just employees. You are partners in the mission. I do not take your commitment for granted.

To my patients —all of you, every single one. You are the reason this book exists. You walked into my clinic at your most vulnerable, trusted me with your bodies and your fears, and then showed me what human beings are capable of when they refuse to give up. You taught me as much as I taught you —possibly more. The stories woven through these chapters, the victories I describe, the transformations I have been privileged to witness—they are yours. I have simply been honored to be in the room when they happened. You will always be my greatest teachers.

To my Parkinson's Boxing Champions—I call you that because you are. Every session, you show up and you fight—not just for your physical function, but for your dignity, your independence, and your joy. You have grown this program from a small beginning into something I am enormously proud of, and you have done it by choosing, again and again, to believe in what is possible. I am so proud of each of you. Keep fighting. Keep moving. The world needs your example.

To my community—the clients, the podcast listeners, the social media followers, the women who have found their way to my page at 3am looking for answers, and the professionals who have reached out from across the country to say that what I teach has resonated with them. You gave me the courage to write this book by showing me that the message matters. I wrote every chapter with your faces in mind.

To The Bahamas—the island that shaped me. My love of movement, my competitive spirit, my belief that hard work and commitment produce results—all of it was forged there. Track and field days, primary school, junior high, high school—those years built a foundation that has held through everything life has placed on top of it. I carry those roots with me wherever I go.

And finally—to you, the reader. You did not have to pick up this book. You chose to. That choice tells me something important about you: you are ready. You are done settling for less than your best. You are willing to do the work. I wrote every word of this book for the person sitting exactly where you are right now — and I am honored beyond measure that it found its way into your hands.

Now go live it.

With deep gratitude and unwavering belief in your best life,

Dr. Paulette Lewis, DPT
Doctor of Neurological Physical Therapy
Health & Wellness Coach | Consultant | Educator

TABLE OF CONTENTS

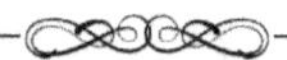

Preface

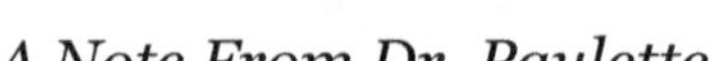

A Note From Dr. Paulette

Welcome. I mean that sincerely—welcome. If you've picked up this book, something in you already knows it's time. Time for more energy. More mental clarity. More confidence in your body and your future. And I want you to know—you are absolutely in the right place.

I'm Dr. Paulette Lewis—a Health and Wellness Coach, consultant, educator, and Doctor of Neurological Physical Therapy with over 26 years of clinical experience. For nine of those years, I've owned and operated my own specialized neurological outpatient therapy clinic, working daily with patients navigating Parkinson's disease, stroke recovery, multiple sclerosis, neuropathy, and the very real challenges of age-related changes in balance and mobility.

I've sat across from hundreds of patients at their most vulnerable —and I have watched them rise. Not because they had perfect circumstances, but because they were given the right tools, the right knowledge, and someone who believed in them fiercely enough to push them toward their own breakthroughs. That's exactly what this book is designed to be for you.

But I want to be honest with you about something: I didn't write this book from a place of having it all figured out. I wrote it from a place of lived experience—as a clinician, yes, but also as a woman in midlife who has personally wrestled with stress, hormonal changes, fatigue, weight gain, disrupted sleep, and the quiet pressure of holding everything together while quietly falling apart on the inside. I've been there.

In some ways, this book is the roadmap I wish someone had handed me. Every chapter in this book is built on decades of clinical research, scientific evidence, and practical strategies—but also on real stories. My stories. My patients' stories. Because information without humanity is just noise. I want you to feel seen in these pages, not just informed.

This book is written for busy professionals, for the aging adult who is finally putting themselves first, and for anyone standing at the crossroads of midlife wondering, *'What now?'* It's for those of you who are done settling for less than your best. Your best life is not behind you. It is waiting — and it starts here.

Let's get to work.

— Dr. Paulette Lewis, DPT

Introduction

Why Mind Strong, Body Strong Works

Let me tell you something about midlife that nobody talks about enough: it is not a decline. It is a pivot point. I know this because I am living it right now. As I write these words, I am squarely in the middle of this season — navigating hormonal shifts, the demands of running a business, the joys and stresses of family life, and the personal work of becoming the healthiest, sharpest, most vibrant version of myself. Midlife has a way of showing you exactly what you've been neglecting, and it does so with zero apologies.

But here's what science confirms, and what I've witnessed in my clinic for over two decades: your brain is adaptable, your body is resilient, and your habits are powerful. The energy dips, the mental fog, the motivation slumps—none of these are life sentences. They are signals. And this book teaches you how to respond to those signals with strategy, not surrender.

The Mind Strong, Body Strong Method is built on four interconnected pillars: ***Nutrition, Movement, Mindset,*** and ***Recovery***. These are not trendy concepts—they are the evidence-backed foundations of how your brain and body work together to either thrive or decline. When you strengthen all four, the results are not just physical. Your thinking sharpens. Your mood lifts. Your confidence returns. Your life expands.

Here is how this book is structured:

- First, you'll understand why your brain is your greatest asset—and how protecting it starts with choices you make every single day.

- Then, you'll build your personal toolkit: fueling your brain with food, strengthening your body through movement, anchoring your motivation with mindset practices, and recharging through intentional recovery.

- Finally, you'll follow a 30-day action plan that integrates all four pillars into real, sustainable habits—with tracking tools and reflection prompts to guide every step.

Each chapter ends with a personal story from my own journey or my clinical work—because I believe deeply that knowing you are not alone in this is half the battle.

After my story, you'll find space for your own reflection, because your story matters too. This is not about perfection. It is not about extreme diets, punishing workouts, or overnight transformation. It is about intentional, consistent action—the kind that compounds quietly over weeks and months until one day you look in the mirror and recognize the version of yourself you've been working toward. Your best life does not require a completely new identity. It requires better information and the courage to apply it. Let's build that together.

CHAPTER 1

Why Your Brain Is Your Superpower

The Mind-Body Connection That Changes Everything

Think about the last time you were truly on your game. Maybe it was a morning when you woke up clear-headed and focused, moved through your to-do list with precision, and felt genuinely energized throughout the day. Or maybe it was a moment in a conversation when your thinking was sharp, your words were right, and you felt fully present. Recall that feeling for just a moment. Now ask yourself: when was the last time you felt that way consistently?

For many people in midlife, that version of themselves feels like a memory. But I want to challenge that story right now, because the science doesn't support it—and neither does my clinical experience.

Your Brain Is the Command Center

Your brain is not just another organ. It is the command center for your entire life—your energy, your focus, your mood, your motivation, and yes, your physical strength and coordination. When your brain is thriving, everything else follows. When it's struggling, even the healthiest diet or most disciplined workout routine feels like pushing a boulder uphill.

One of my favorite things my maternal grandmother used to say was this: *"when you have health and strength, you are rich."* I've thought about those words more times than I can count throughout my career. Because no amount of money, success, or status can purchase genuine neurological health. When the brain isn't functioning well, wealth doesn't feel like wealth at all.

As a Neurological Physical Therapist, I spend my days in the space where brain health and physical function intersect. I treat patients with Parkinson's disease, stroke survivors, people with multiple sclerosis, neuropathy, and complex balance disorders. What I've learned from working with this population—day after day, year after year — is this: the brain's capacity to change, adapt, and improve is far greater than most people realize. We call it neuroplasticity, and it is nothing short of a game-changer.

Why Midlife Is the Critical Window

As we move through our forties and fifties, subtle shifts in brain function begin to surface. Focus isn't quite as sharp. Memory occasionally slips in ways that feel unfamiliar. Motivation requires more effort to summon. Many of my patients describe this as feeling like they're 'not quite themselves,' and for many—especially women navigating perimenopause and menopause—these changes can feel alarming and isolating.

But here's what I need you to hear: these changes are common, but they are not inevitable. They are not a life sentence. The brain remains remarkably adaptable well into midlife and beyond. With targeted strategies — the kind we'll build together throughout this book — you can boost cognition, protect against further decline, and reclaim mental clarity and vitality, which you thought were things you could no longer do.

The Science of Neuroplasticity

Neuroplasticity refers to the brain's ability to reorganize, form new neural connections, and adapt in response to experience, learning, and deliberate practice. In the neurological world, this concept is the foundation of everything we do clinically. It's why a stroke survivor can relearn how to walk. It's why a Parkinson's patient can improve their gait speed and balance with consistent, targeted exercise. And it's why you—regardless of your current state—have the capacity to strengthen your brain starting right now.

Physical activity, quality nutrition, restorative sleep, and an intentional mindset are not 'nice-to-haves' in this equation. They are the direct inputs that drive neuroplasticity. Every step you take, every nourishing meal you eat, every night of quality sleep you prioritize—these are investments directly into the health and performance of your brain.

The Brain-Body Connection Is Not a Theory

In my clinic, I don't just treat bodies. I treat the whole person—brain, body, and mindset together. Many of my patients come in expecting physical exercises, and they get that. But they also get education. They get mental imagery training. They get taught about the power of their own beliefs, the role of nutrition in nervous system function, and the importance of sleep in neurological recovery. Because I learned early in my career that when you ignore the mind-body connection, you leave the most powerful tool on the table.

Treating your brain as the ultimate performance tool isn't arrogance—it's accuracy. When you do, the results ripple outward: clearer decisions, steadier energy, greater resilience under stress, and a body that moves with more confidence and less pain. That is what this book is designed to help you build. One chapter at a time, one habit at a time.

From My Journey To Yours

As a Neurological Physical Therapist, my days have always been centered around the brain and nervous system. But I'll be honest—it wasn't until 2025 that something shifted in how I approached my patients. My thinking moved from *'How do I treat this patient?'* to *'How do I teach this patient to treat themselves?'* That shift changed everything in my practice. I began focusing more intentionally on helping people recognize the direct, tangible connection between their minds and their bodies—and more importantly, on teaching them how to use that connection as a therapeutic tool.

One patient stands out vividly in my mind. I'll call her **'V'** to protect her privacy. V had come to me previously for gait and balance issues, and she'd made real progress. But then she fell, and that fall set her back considerably—not just physically, but mentally. She came back to me using a front-wheeled walker, when before the fall she'd been walking with a single-point cane. Her goal was to return to that cane. We worked hard together. Her physical strength improved. Her gait mechanics got better. But there was a ceiling she kept hitting, and I couldn't figure out why— until one session, when it became clear. It wasn't her body that was holding her back. It was her mind. Specifically, her fear of falling again.

In physical therapy school, we study psychology—and I can honestly say that earning an 'A' in that course paid dividends I didn't fully appreciate at the time. I drew on that training here. V and I began using mental imagery: before every gait training session, we spent time having her visualize herself walking upright, balanced, and confident—exactly as she had before the fall. We worked on releasing the fear and reconnecting her conscious mind with the muscle memory her body already had stored.

The breakthrough was remarkable. Once we addressed the mental block, V's physical progress accelerated rapidly. She met her goal. She left that clinic walking with a cane—upright, confident, and free from the fear that had been limiting her far more than any physical deficit ever had. Her mind and body had always been connected. We just had to remind them of that.

Your Turn To Reflect

Think of a moment in your own life when you realized your mind and body were more connected than you thought. What triggered that awareness—and how did it shift the way you approached your health, your recovery, or your daily choices? Write freely below.

____

____

____

____

____

____

____

CHAPTER 2

—⁓⁓—

The Neuro Wellness Blueprint

Midlife Reimagined — Your Roadmap to Activation

If Chapter 1 convinced you that your brain is your superpower, then Chapter 2 is where you learn how to activate it. This is your roadmap—a practical, science-backed framework for strengthening your mind and body simultaneously. I call it the Mind Strong, Body Strong Method, and it is built on three foundational pillars: ***Nutrition, Movement,*** and ***Mindset***.

I want to be clear about what this framework is and what it isn't. It is not a fad program. It is not a 30-day quick fix designed to fade after the calendar flips. It's a lifestyle architecture — one built on evidence, personal experience, and the clinical wisdom of over two decades of neurological rehabilitation practice.

• Pillar 1: Fuel Your Brain and Body — Nutrition

What you eat directly impacts your energy, your focus, your mood, and your long-term neurological health. Yet the nutrition landscape is noisier than it has ever been. Every week there seems to be a new diet, a new superfood, a new miracle supplement. People want your attention, and frankly, they want your money. I understand the confusion—I navigated it myself.

So let's cut through the noise and return to what the research consistently supports: a foundation built on nutrient-dense whole foods, strategic hydration, brain-supportive nutrients, and balanced blood sugar throughout the day. That's it. Not a program with a trademark. Not a list of foods to fear. A return to intentional, intelligent eating.

- Prioritize colorful vegetables, lean proteins, healthy fats, and whole grains at every meal.

- Omega-3 fatty acids, antioxidants, and B-vitamins are your brain's best allies.

- Hydration is non-negotiable. Even mild dehydration impairs cognition and energy.

- Timing matters: balanced meals every 3–4 hours prevent the blood sugar crashes that derail focus and motivation.

Action Step

Start a food and energy log for three days. Record your meals, snacks, hydration, and energy levels throughout each day. Look for the patterns: when are you sharpest? When do you crash? What did you eat before each? This awareness is your starting point.

- **Pillar 2: Move Your Body, Strengthen Your Brain — Exercise & Mobility**

Your body is not simply a vessel that carries your brain around. It is the engine that powers it. Every step, stretch, and strength exercise you perform sends signals directly to your brain — stimulating neuroplasticity, improving oxygen flow, releasing growth factors that support cognition and mood. I teach this in my clinic every single day. I also live it personally.

Exercise is not a vanity project for me—it is a clinical intervention. And the evidence is clear: regular physical movement is one of the most powerful things you can do for neurological health, cardiovascular function, metabolic health, and emotional well-being.

- Strength training preserves muscle mass, protects joints, and supports metabolism.

- Cardiovascular movement drives oxygen to the brain and stimulates neurogenesis — the actual growth of new brain cells.

- Daily mobility and flexibility work reduces stiffness, improves posture, and prevents the injuries that sideline people for weeks or months.

- Consistency over intensity: 20–30 minutes of intentional movement daily does more for your brain and body than sporadic hard workouts.

Action Step

Schedule at least 20 minutes of movement for each of the next five days. Mix it up—include some strength, some mobility, and something you genuinely enjoy. Log how you feel before and after. Notice the pattern.

- **Pillar 3: Train Your Mind — Mindset & Motivation**

Here is a truth that I have repeated in every speaking engagement, every patient consultation, and every coaching session I have ever led: if your mindset isn't right, the other two pillars will eventually crumble. Motivation is a finite resource. Mindset is a trainable skill — and it is the difference between the person who sustains transformation and the one who cycles through programs year after year without lasting change.

Daily reflection, visualization, and intentional goal-setting are not soft suggestions. They are neurologically grounded practices that prime your brain for the behaviors you want to build. We'll go deep on this in Chapter 4.

- Five minutes of morning reflection to set intention and priorities creates neurological focus for the entire day.

- Visualization — truly imagining yourself achieving your goals — activates the same neural pathways as the behavior itself.

- Celebrating small wins reinforces the dopamine-driven reward cycles that make habits stick.

Action Step

Each morning this week, write down one small health-related action you will complete that day. Not a long list — just one. Track your completion rate. You may be surprised how this simple practice builds momentum.

The Synergy of All Three Pillars

The beauty of this method is that the pillars amplify each other. Proper nutrition fuels your workouts. Movement stimulates your brain. Mindset ensures you keep showing up. You don't have to perfect all three simultaneously — start where you are, apply what you can, and build from there. The compound effect of consistent effort across all three pillars is nothing short of transformative.

From My Journey To Yours

When I opened my clinic, I was excited. I had dreamed of being a business owner, had worked toward it for years, and finally, it was real. What I was not prepared for was the stress that came with it. Growing a business while being a full-time clinician, a wife, and a mother of two active children— it was a load I had underestimated. My business partner was not clinical, which meant the full weight of patient care, clinical documentation, staff management, and local operations fell entirely on me. Sleep became a casualty. Exercise got pushed to the back burner. The weight started to creep up. And then my blood pressure followed.

"Hypertension." In my family, that word carries weight. My maternal grandmother died from her second stroke. My parents both had high blood pressure. My entire adult life, I had been determined to break that pattern. Yet here I was, being told by my physician that I needed medication. That was my turning

point. Not because of pride—but because I finally stopped and asked myself the honest question: *What am I doing to myself?* I could not keep burning the candle at both ends and expect a different outcome. So, I made changes. Real ones.

I got back to the gym. I cleaned up my nutrition. I became a solo business owner and reclaimed a level of control over my own schedule. I started treating my own health with the same intentionality I brought to my patients' care. And the blood pressure came down. The energy came back. The clarity returned. I became the example I had been asking my patients to become — and my lived experience became the foundation of everything you're reading in this book.

Your Turn To Reflect

Describe a time in your own midlife when a challenge forced you to re-evaluate your priorities. What shifted — in your health, your habits, your perspective — and what new direction opened up as a result? Use the space below to explore that turning point.

____

____

____

____

____

____

CHAPTER 3

Nutrition for Brain Power

The Power of Neuroplasticity on Your Plate

If your brain is your superpower, then food is the fuel that either ignites it or extinguishes it. What you eat every single day has a direct and measurable effect on your cognitive function, your energy stability, your mood regulation, and your long-term neurological health. This is not wellness theory—this is neuroscience.

Your brain consumes approximately 20% of the calories you take in each day—remarkable, given that it represents only about 2% of your total body weight. It is the most metabolically expensive organ you have, and it is relentlessly demanding. When you feed it processed foods, excess sugar, and refined carbohydrates, you are essentially putting cheap gasoline in a high-performance engine. The initial effect might feel like energy — but it is followed quickly by crashes, brain fog, inflammation, and over time, the kind of cognitive decline we once wrote off as 'just getting older.'

I'll tell you plainly: as a healthcare provider, I am deeply aware of how much the healthcare industry financially benefits from poor dietary choices. Poor nutrition is a driver of chronic disease, and chronic disease keeps clinics full. I am not in this to keep you sick. I am in this to help you thrive — and that starts with what's on your plate

What Your Brain Needs Most

Through both my clinical work and my personal pursuit of nutritional education—including a nutritional certification I was completing at the time of this writing—I have identified the nutrients that matter most for midlife brain health:

- **Found in salmon, sardines, chia seeds, and walnuts —** support memory function and neuroplasticity. Omega-3 fatty acids

- **From berries, leafy greens, and colorful vegetables —** fight oxidative stress and brain inflammation. Antioxidants

- **From eggs, leafy greens, and fortified whole grains —** support energy metabolism and mood regulation. B-vitamins

- **From fish, poultry, legumes, and beans —** sustains energy and supports neurotransmitter production. Lean protein

- **Found abundantly in eggs**—supports memory and brain cell communication, both of which tend to decline in midlife. Choline

- Protect the brain against oxidative stress and inflammation, and vitamin D specifically plays a role in preventing cognitive decline. Vitamins C, D, and E, plus selenium

Stabilizing Energy: The Midlife Balancing Act

Blood sugar instability is one of the most underappreciated contributors to midlife fatigue, brain fog, and mood swings. When energy crashes mid-morning or mid-afternoon, willpower evaporates—and with it, the motivation to move, to make good food choices, and to show up fully in your day.

- Eat every 3–4 hours to prevent blood sugar crashes and maintain consistent mental energy.

- Include protein at every meal to support neurotransmitter production and sustained focus.

- Choose smart carbohydrates — whole grains, fruits, legumes — over refined sugars and processed snacks.

- Hydrate consistently. Aim for at least 2 liters of water daily. Dehydration impairs memory, attention, and cognitive processing.

Quick Start Tip

Start your day with a breakfast that includes protein, healthy fat, and complex carbohydrates — like Greek yogurt with berries and chia seeds, or eggs with whole-grain toast and avocado. This combination sets your brain up for sustained focus and stable energy from the first hour of the day. It also supports healthy gut function — and emerging research makes it increasingly clear that gut health directly influences brain function and mental well-being.

Anti-Inflammatory Eating for Brain Longevity

Neuroinflammation — chronic, low-grade inflammation in the brain — is increasingly recognized as a driver of cognitive decline, including in conditions like Parkinson's disease and Alzheimer's. Research by Sartori and colleagues (2012) confirmed that neuroinflammation can cause memory loss, slowed brain processing, and confusion. The good news: diet is one of our most powerful tools for managing inflammation.

Top anti-inflammatory foods to prioritize:

- Fatty fish: salmon, mackerel, sardines
- Dark leafy greens: spinach, kale, arugula
- Berries: blueberries, strawberries, raspberries
- Nuts and seeds: almonds, walnuts, flaxseed
- Anti-inflammatory spices: turmeric, ginger, cinnamon

Mindful Eating: Awareness as a Practice

Eating isn't just a biological function—it's an act of intention. Mindful eating means slowing down, recognizing true hunger versus emotional cravings, and actually tasting and appreciating the food you're consuming. It improves digestion, reduces overeating, and creates a positive relationship with food that sustains long-term change.

A simple practice: before each meal, pause for three deep breaths. Notice your hunger level. Take your first few bites slowly and with full attention. This small shift, practiced consistently, can meaningfully change your relationship with food—and by extension, your energy and cognitive performance.

From My Journey To Yours

I have loved talking about nutrition since junior high school. That curiosity led me to pursue a nutritional certification—because as a physical therapist and neurological specialist, I needed to be able to speak intelligently to my patients about how the food they were eating was affecting the very conditions I was treating.

Two patients stand out most vividly when I think about the power of nutritional change. Both were women. Both were coming to my clinic around the same time for neurological PT services—one dealing with the complications of neuropathy, the other managing multiple sclerosis. Both were overweight, and one was approaching the threshold of obesity. I knew immediately that movement was going to be laborious for both of them, not just because of their neurological diagnoses, but because of the additional physical burden their weight was placing on already-compromised nervous systems. I also knew I had a professional and moral responsibility to have the conversation—gently, but honestly.

I educated each of them on research-based dietary approaches that were specific to their diagnoses—not to prescribe a diet, but to equip them with information they could explore and implement on their own terms. I trusted them to make their own choices. And they did.

Months later, both women returned to my clinic for follow-up care. The transformation was visible before either of them said a word. Significant weight loss. Brighter eyes. A confidence in how they carried themselves that hadn't been there before. One of them— the patient who had first arrived in a wheelchair—walked into my clinic under her own power, without even a cane. She didn't need one anymore. Nutrition did that. Not me. I simply gave them the information and the belief that it was possible. They did the rest. And I will never forget either of them.

Your Turn To Reflect

Reflect on a time when a change in how you ate — or how you thought about food — made a noticeable difference in how you felt physically or mentally. What was the shift, and what did it teach you about the relationship between what you consume and how you function? Write your reflection below.

CHAPTER 4

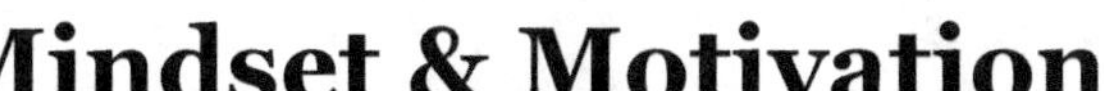

Mindset & Motivation

Stress, Resilience, and the Mental Game of Thriving

You've built the nutritional foundation. You understand why your brain needs to be protected and fueled. But without the right mindset, all the best intentions in the world will eventually yield to the pressure of a busy day, a stressful week, or the relentless pull of old habits. Mindset is not a soft skill — it is the master lever. And in midlife especially, stress and inflammation are working against it.

The connection between chronic stress, neurological inflammation, and cognitive decline is well established. Cortisol — the primary stress hormone — when chronically elevated, directly impairs memory, disrupts sleep, promotes fat storage, and compromises immune function. The brain under prolonged stress is not operating at its potential. It is surviving. And thriving requires something different.

Why Mindset Changes the Brain

In the neurological world, motor imagery and mental imagery are well-recognized therapeutic tools. When a patient visualizes performing a movement—truly sees and feels it in their mind's eye—the brain activates the same neural pathways involved in executing that movement. This is neuroplasticity in action. Thought patterns, practiced consistently, physically reshape the brain. I've used this technique with Parkinson's patients. I've used it with stroke survivors. And I've used it in my own life. The stories you tell yourself—about who you are, what you're capable of, what you deserve—are being literally encoded into your brain's wiring.

That means the inverse is also true: you can choose different thoughts, practice them deliberately, and over time, rewire your response patterns.

The Three Pillars of a Thriving Mindset

1. Self-Awareness

Self-awareness is the foundation. Without it, you cannot identify the thought patterns that are holding you back, the habits that are draining your energy, or the emotional triggers that lead you away from your goals. Something as small as 15 extra minutes in the morning—before you check your phone, before the household wakes up—spent quietly in reflection can change the entire trajectory of your day.

2. Positive Reinforcement

Progress requires celebration — even the small stuff. Did you drink your water today? Take a brisk walk at lunch? Choose grilled over fried? That is progress. And your brain needs to hear that it is. Positive reinforcement activates dopamine pathways that make the behavior more likely to repeat. We are wired to continue what feels rewarding. Use that to your advantage.

3. Visualization and Goal Clarity

Mental imagery is not just motivational—it is physiological. When you vividly picture yourself completing your goals—your energy, your posture, your confidence, your capability—your brain begins laying the neural groundwork for that reality. Make visualization a daily practice: a few minutes each morning or evening, seeing your best self clearly and with full sensory detail.

Building Motivation That Outlasts the Feeling

Motivation is an emotion—and like all emotions, it fluctuates. Building a healthy life on the back of motivation alone is like building a house on sand. What you need underneath motivation are habits, structure, and accountability. Here's how to build them:

- **Start small.** Start with one or two habits at a time. Success creates momentum. Overwhelm creates paralysis.

- **Stack habits onto existing routines.** Attach new behaviors to things you already do consistently — exercise after your morning coffee, prep your lunch while dinner cooks.

- **Track progress visually.** Seeing progress is itself motivating. Use a journal, a simple checklist, or an app to track daily wins.

- **Build an accountability system.** One person, a group, a coach — it doesn't matter the size of the village. Having someone who holds you accountable changes everything.

Action Step

Write one health-related goal for this week in your journal. Beside it, write one small, specific daily action that moves you toward it. Review it each morning. Check it off each evening. Watch what that simple practice does to your focus and follow-through over seven days.

From My Journey To Yours

Between 2023 and 2024, stress arrived at my door in a way I had not anticipated. My husband—an only child—became the sole caretaker for his father after two brain bleeds and two surgeries. He was out of town for weeks, sometimes months at a time. Simultaneously, I was managing a growing clinical practice, raising our son through high school, supporting our daughter through her first year of college, and navigating the early stages of perimenopause without fully understanding what was happening to my body.

I was fatigued. Anxious. Struggling with sleep disruptions I had never experienced before. Weight gain seemed to appear out of nowhere and wouldn't budge. So did the kind of low-grade depression that doesn't announce itself dramatically—it just quietly dims your light. And I was supposed to be the one keeping everything together. Because research and learning are deeply part of who I am, I turned to podcasts and research reading. I found a symptom checklist for perimenopause and started checking boxes—too many of them. That recognition alone was a turning point. Naming what was happening gave me the power to address it.

I started journaling again—something I hadn't made time for in years. It became a lifeline for processing the anxiety and quieting the mental noise. I returned to my happy places: the gym, the bookstore, my church. I implemented nutritional changes and began using targeted supplementation to support my brain. I put a cognitive plan together for myself—the same kind of plan I had been building for patients.

Slowly, the balance returned. The sleep improved. The weight started moving again. And perhaps most importantly, I started to feel like myself again. My lived experience became one of the most powerful clinical tools I have—because now when I sit across from a patient or client who is drowning under stress, I can speak from the inside out. I know what it feels like to be depleted. And I know what it takes to come back.

Your Turn To Reflect

Describe a season when chronic stress—from work, caregiving, health challenges, or life transitions—began to impact your physical or mental performance. How did you recognize the signs, and what strategies helped you regain your footing? Use the space below to reflect on your own resilience story.

____

____

____

CHAPTER 5

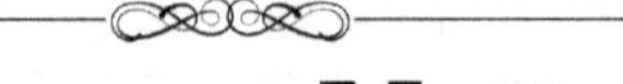

Movement Matters

Movement as Medicine — The Engine That Powers It All

If nutrition fuels your brain and mindset sustains your consistency, then movement is the engine that drives transformation into your body. You were built to move. Every joint, every muscle, every neurological pathway in your body is designed for motion—and when that motion becomes restricted by sedentary habits, stress, or the quiet accumulation of age-related changes, the cascade effect touches every system you have.

Here is something that often surprises people: physical therapists are movement specialists. Not just rehabilitation specialists—movement specialists. Our education and clinical training equip us to analyze, prescribe, and optimize movement not only for people recovering from injuries or managing disease, but for healthy individuals seeking to perform better, age more gracefully, and prevent the very conditions that fill my clinic's schedule. If we can help you recover from an injury, we can absolutely help you prevent one in the first place.

Why Movement Is Neurologically Essential

Exercise does far more than shape the body. It is one of the most potent neurological interventions available to us:

- It increases cerebral blood flow, directly supporting memory, attention, and cognitive processing speed.

- It triggers the release of BDNF—Brain-Derived Neurotrophic Factor—which promotes the growth of new neurons and strengthens existing neural connections.

- It reduces cortisol and inflammatory markers, creating a brain environment more hospitable to learning and recovery.

- It improves sleep quality, which is a cornerstone of neurological repair and consolidation.

Complex, coordinated movements specifically stimulate neuroplasticity—which is why activities like boxing, dance, and resistance training are so valuable for neurological patients.

The Three Types of Movement You Need

1. Strength Training

Muscle mass naturally declines with age—a process called *sarcopenia*—and with it goes metabolism, joint stability, posture, and functional independence. Strength training reverses this process. It protects your joints, supports your metabolic health, and fortifies the foundation of your physical capability. You do not need a gym membership or heavy equipment to begin. Bodyweight squats, push-ups, resistance band rows, and glute bridges are powerful, effective, and accessible from anywhere.

2. Cardiovascular Movement

Cardio is your brain's oxygen delivery system. Whether it's brisk walking, cycling, swimming, or high-intensity interval training, the goal is elevating your heart rate into a range where physiological adaptation occurs. For Parkinson's patients, research supports exercising at 60–80% of maximum heart rate for optimal dopamine receptor stimulation. For all of us, the same range drives cardiovascular adaptation, weight management, and neuroplasticity. If you can find a friend or group to move with, even better—the social component increases consistency and adds what researchers call the *Köhler effect: we push harder in the presence of others.*

3. Mobility and Flexibility

This is the component most people skip—and it is the one that comes back to haunt them. As we age, joint mobility and soft tissue flexibility are among the first things to erode. Rounded shoulders, forward head posture, tight hips, stiff ankles—these are patterns I see daily in my clinic, and they are almost entirely preventable with consistent, intentional mobility work. Even five minutes a day of targeted stretching and movement makes a measurable difference over weeks and months. Your future self will thank you.

Building Your Movement Practice

Start where you are, not where you think you should be. Here is a simple, sustainable framework:

- **Daily Movement:** 20–30 minutes minimum. A brisk walk, a short strength circuit, or a yoga session—the key is daily habit, not daily intensity.

- **Strength Training:** 2–3 sessions per week. Focus on major muscle groups. Use bodyweight, resistance bands, or hand weights depending on what is available to you.

- **Mobility Practice:** Daily. Every morning or evening, five to ten minutes of targeted stretching and rolling. This is non-negotiable as you move through midlife.

Action Step

Schedule three 'movement appointments' in your calendar this week. Treat them as non-negotiable commitments — the same way you would a meeting with someone else. After each session, log your energy level, mood, and any physical observations. The data you gather about your own body is invaluable.

From My Journey To Yours

Anyone who knows me knows that exercise is not a chore to me — it is a calling. I have loved movement since I was a child in The Bahamas, running track, playing sports, and finding every opportunity to be active. That love carried me through my undergraduate years, where I seriously considered athletic training and sports medicine before finding my true clinical home in neurological physical therapy.

I bring that passion into my practice every single day. Neuro patients face unique challenges—their diagnoses are complex, often progressive, and rarely curable. But the reward of working with this population comes from exactly that challenge. And movement is always at the center of their rehabilitation.

I had one patient—I'll call him Mr. Y—who arrived with a Parkinson's diagnosis. We worked together diligently, and while he did show improvement, there was a ceiling we couldn't break through. His gains were inconsistent, and something wasn't adding up clinically. I advocated for further testing. The result revealed a different diagnosis entirely: normal pressure hydrocephalus (NPH) — a condition whose symptoms can closely mimic Parkinson's disease.

Once Mr. Y received the appropriate intervention—a shunt placement—everything changed. He had been a bodybuilder in a previous chapter of his life. His single biggest goal when he first walked into my clinic was to get back to the gym. After his surgery, with the therapeutic plan I built for him and the work he put in, we actually went to the gym together—his clinic graduation, in a sense. I watched him lift weights again. I watched him return to something that had defined him, that he thought he'd lost forever.

That day reminded me why movement matters beyond the physical. It restores identity. It rebuilds dignity. It gives people back something that was taken from them. Movement is medicine—but it is also meaning.

Your Turn To Reflect

Share a moment when movement — whether exercise, therapy, or simply getting back to a physical activity you loved — transformed something for you or someone you know. What was the barrier? What was the breakthrough? Use the space below to capture that story.

____

____

____

____

____

____

CHAPTER 6

Strength & Mobility

Strength and Longevity — Non-Negotiables for Midlife

Let me be direct with you: strength training is not optional for midlife longevity. It is one of the single most impactful investments you can make in your future health, independence, and quality of life. I do not say this as a fitness enthusiast— though I am one. I say it as a clinician who spends her days working with people whose functional independence has been compromised, and who can trace many of those challenges directly back to years of insufficient strength and mobility work.

Strong muscles are not just about aesthetics. They stabilize joints, protect against injury, support metabolic function, and— critically for neurological health—reduce fall risk. Flexible, mobile joints reduce pain, improve posture, and allow your body to move efficiently through all of the demands of daily life. Together, strength and mobility are the physical foundation upon which everything else is built.

Core Principles of Midlife Strength Training

- **Consistency over intensity.** Short, regular sessions outperform sporadic, exhausting ones. Even two to three 20-minute sessions weekly produces meaningful results over time.

- **Functional movement first.** Focus on exercises that mimic real-life actions — squatting, reaching, carrying, bending. These build the functional strength that actually improves daily living.

- **Progressive overload.** Gradually increase resistance, reps, or complexity to continue challenging your muscles and nervous system. This is how you prevent plateaus.

- **Balance and control.** Controlled movements engage stabilizing muscles, protect joints, and reduce injury risk. Form before weight — always.

Essential Strength Exercises by Category

- **Lower Body**

1. **Bodyweight Squats** — strengthen quadriceps, hamstrings, and glutes.

2. **Step-Ups** — improve single-leg strength and balance.

3. **Glute Bridges** — target the glutes and lower back while protecting the spine.

- **Upper Body**

1. **Push-Ups (or Wall Push-Ups)** — build chest, shoulder, and arm strength.

2. **Resistance Band Rows** — strengthen the back and counteract the forward-rounded posture so prevalent in midlife.

3. **Shoulder Press** — improve upper body stability and overhead reach capability.

- **Core**

1. **Planks** — Train the entire core including the deep stabilizers that protect your spine.

2. **Dead Bugs** — Engage deep core muscles with coordination and breath control.

3. **Russian Twists** — Build rotational strength for functional everyday movements.

Action Step

Choose 3–4 exercises from each category above. Begin with 2–3 sets of 8–12 repetitions, focusing entirely on form before adding any additional load. Schedule these sessions two to three times per week, and track your progress. You will be surprised how quickly your body responds.

Mobility: The Other Half of the Equation

In my clinic, I hear patients say they feel 'stiff' before almost anything else. Stiffness in the hips, neck, shoulders, and ankles is one of the earliest signs that mobility work is being neglected—and one of the most preventable sources of pain and functional limitation.

- **Hip Circles and Leg Swings** improve hip joint mobility and warm up the entire lower chain.

- **Cat-Cow Stretch** loosens the thoracic and lumbar spine and counters the effects of prolonged sitting.

- **Chest Opener Stretch** addresses the rounded shoulder posture that develops from desk work and forward-facing daily habits.

- **Ankle Circles** support balance, gait stability, and fall prevention.

A practical framework: Begin every training session with 5–10 minutes of dynamic mobility to prepare your joints. Follow with your strength work. Close with static stretching for flexibility and recovery. This sequence is not just good programming—it's injury prevention architecture.

From My Journey To Yours

Exercise has been part of my identity since childhood. I was the Tomboy who climbed poles, ran track, and found any excuse to be moving. That love for athletics followed me into college, into my professional life, and eventually into the Parkinson's Boxing program I created as an extension of my neurological clinic.

Strength training specifically has been part of my life since university—and it remains so today. I lift weights because I know, clinically and personally, that the muscle you build in your forties directly influences the quality of your life in your sixties, seventies, and beyond. I see this truth every day in my patients.

When I started my boxing program, I began with one woman and two men. None of them had ever boxed before. Most had never considered that they could do something physically demanding given their Parkinson's diagnosis. There's often a misconception that a program called 'boxing' means fighting — it does not. What it means is high-intensity, neurologically stimulating movement that research shows is particularly beneficial for people with Parkinson's disease, helping reduce symptom progression and promote neuroplasticity.

I did not shy away from making my participants work hard. That was intentional. They needed to understand that they were capable of more than their diagnosis suggested. And when they experienced that for themselves—when they felt their own strength, their own capability—the transformation was not just physical. Their posture changed. Their confidence changed. Their belief in themselves changed.

My foundational crew—those first three members—are still with me years later. They have become my most enthusiastic advocates. And they remind me, every session, why strength is not optional. It is the thing that keeps people in their own lives, on their own terms, for as long as possible.

Your Turn To Reflect

Think of a moment when you—or someone you care about—realized that building strength was not optional, but essential. What sparked that realization? What changed as a result? Reflect on your relationship with physical strength, and what it means to you now, in the space below.

____

____

____

____

____

____

CHAPTER 7

Recovery & Energy Management

Nutrition for Brain and Body — Rest as a Neurological Tool

There is a habit of thought in our culture that equates constant productivity with value. Rest gets labeled as laziness. Downtime is something to feel guilty about. And recovery—the deliberate act of restoring your nervous system, your muscles, and your mental reserves—is treated as optional. It is not optional. It is strategic. And nowhere is this more true than in midlife, when the body's tolerance for chronic stress, sleep deprivation, and neglected recovery narrows significantly.

Recovery is what allows your nutrition to actually work. It is what allows your movement to translate into strength and neurological adaptation rather than fatigue and breakdown. Without adequate recovery, even the most perfectly designed nutrition and exercise plan will plateau—and eventually, it will cause harm.

The Three Pillars of Recovery

1. Sleep: The Master Restorer

Sleep is the most powerful neurological recovery tool available to us—and it is largely free. During deep sleep, the brain consolidates memories, processes emotional experiences, clears metabolic waste products through the glymphatic system, and repairs the neurological structures that cognition and movement depend on. Aim for 7–9 hours per night. Consistency matters as much as duration—your body and brain perform best on a predictable circadian rhythm.

- Keep a consistent bedtime and wake time, even on weekends.

- Limit screen exposure for 60 minutes before bed. Blue light suppresses melatonin production.

- Keep your room dark, cool, and quiet. These environmental conditions support the sleep architecture your brain needs.

2. Active Recovery

Recovery does not always mean stillness. Gentle movement on rest days—walking, light cycling, yoga, foam rolling—enhances circulation, reduces delayed-onset muscle soreness, and maintains the neurological patterns your training is building. The goal is low intensity and intentional ease, not another hard session in disguise.

3. Stress Management and Nervous System Regulation

Chronic psychological stress is one of the most effective destroyers of recovery quality there is. When cortisol remains elevated, sleep suffers, inflammation rises, tissue repair slows, and the motivational circuitry of the brain becomes increasingly difficult to activate. Managing stress is not a luxury—it is a physiological necessity.

- Deep, diaphragmatic breathing activates the parasympathetic nervous system—your body's 'rest and repair' mode—within minutes.

- Meditation and mindfulness practices reduce cortisol, improve emotional regulation, and strengthen the prefrontal cortex over time.

- Journaling externalizes mental clutter, reduces rumination, and creates space for genuine mental rest.

Nutritional Support for Recovery

What you eat in the hours surrounding your training sessions and sleep directly impacts how well you recover. Protein intake in the post-exercise window supports muscle repair. Magnesium-rich foods—leafy greens, nuts, seeds—support nervous system relaxation and sleep quality. Consistent hydration throughout the day maintains the cellular conditions your recovery depends on. Avoid heavy meals and alcohol close to bedtime—both interfere with sleep architecture and neurological restoration.

Action Step

This week, track three things daily: your sleep duration and quality, your energy level at three points in the day (morning, midday, evening), and which recovery strategies you used. At the end of the week, look for the patterns. The data you gather about your own body is the foundation of a truly personalized recovery plan.

From My Journey To Yours

My colleague, Dr. Katrina Banks, DPT, and I host a collaborative podcast called Neurowellness Conversations. On more than one occasion, we've talked about rest and energy—and her message is one I've taken deeply to heart: *rest is power.* As a woman who transitioned into menopause during the writing of this book, I can speak to this topic with considerable personal authority. Before menopause, I was a workhorse in the gym. I ran a clinic, raised a family, built a business, and powered through most things on energy and drive. Sleep was something I fit in around everything else.

Menopause corrected that thinking very quickly. The hot flashes, the disrupted sleep, the anxious nights, the unexplained fatigue—none of it responded to the same strategies that had always worked for me before. I had to start from a new understanding of my own body.

I began going to bed at a consistent hour—not when the work was done, but at an actual time I committed to. I invested in blackout curtains and cooled the room. I stopped scrolling through social media or answering emails in the late evening. I had real conversations with my husband—a self-described night owl and my better half—about what my sleep environment needed to look like. That wasn't always easy, but it was necessary. His help was a key to my successful changes. These changes worked. Sleep improved.

Cortisol began to normalize. The weight started to respond again. The cognitive sharpness I had felt slipping came back. I share this not to offer my routine as the prescription, but to offer it as evidence: rest is not weakness. It is where recovery happens. It is where your brain consolidates what you've learned, repairs what exercise has built, and prepares you to show up fully for another day. If you've been treating sleep as negotiable, I want to invite you—strongly—to reconsider that.

Your Turn To Reflect

Think of a time when depleted energy— from poor sleep, overwork, hormonal changes, or chronic stress—impacted your physical or mental performance. What ultimately helped you restore your vitality? What was the turning point? Use the space below to trace your own energy story.

____

____

____

____

CHAPTER 8

Habits That Last

Energy, Discipline, and the Architecture of Lasting Change

Knowledge is not transformation. I want to say that clearly, because it is one of the most important truths in this book. You can read every wellness resource ever written, understand the biochemistry of neuroplasticity, and have a nutrition plan drawn up by the best registered dietitian in the country—and none of it will change your life until you build the habits that make those things real, consistent, and automatic.

Habits are the infrastructure of the life you want. They are the daily architecture of your health, your energy, and your performance. Motivation gets you started. Discipline carries you through the days when motivation has gone quiet. And habits are what remain after discipline stops requiring effort—when the good choice becomes the default choice.

Why Habits Outperform Motivation in Midlife

Motivation is an emotional state. It rises and falls with circumstances, sleep quality, hormonal fluctuations, stress levels, and the weather. It is completely unreliable as a foundation for sustained behavior change—and never more so than in midlife, when the physiological landscape is actively shifting.

Habits, by contrast, are automatic behaviors. They don't require deliberation, willpower, or inspiration. The more you structure your environment and routines to make healthy behaviors the path of least resistance, the less you have to rely on how you feel in any given moment. Think of habits as outsourcing your decisions to your past, best self.

The Habit-Building Blueprint

• Start Small and Stay Consistent

The most common mistake people make when beginning a new health regimen is attempting too much change at once. The result is overwhelm, unsustainability, and eventual abandonment. Instead, choose one habit in each pillar and commit to it fully for two to three weeks before adding another. Small, consistent action always outperforms ambitious, sporadic effort.

• Stack New Habits onto Existing Ones

Habit stacking leverages the neural grooves of your existing routines. Attach a new behavior to something you already do automatically: after your morning coffee, do five minutes of mobility work. After brushing your teeth, drink a full glass of water. After you close your laptop for the day, take a ten-minute walk. The existing habit acts as the trigger; the new one rides in on its coattails.

• Use Environmental Design

Your environment either supports your habits or sabotages them. Resistance bands visible by your desk, a water bottle on your nightstand, healthy snacks at eye level in the refrigerator—these small environmental modifications reduce friction and make the healthy choice the easy choice.

• Track Progress and Celebrate Every Win

Visual tracking—a simple journal, a calendar checkmark, an app — makes progress tangible and reinforces the neural reward pathways that sustain motivation. Equally important is celebrating wins, regardless of size. Did you move for 20 minutes today? That is a win. Chose water over soda? That is a win. The brain learns to repeat what it experiences as rewarding. Give it the signal.

- **Focus on Systems, Not Just Goals**

Goals give you direction. Systems create momentum. Instead of 'I want to lose 15 pounds,' build the system: move 30 minutes daily, include protein at every meal, prioritize 7–8 hours of sleep. When the system is functioning, the outcomes follow naturally.

Action Step

Choose one habit from each pillar this week — one from nutrition, one from movement, one from mindset. Track each one daily. At the end of the week, review: which stuck easily, and which required effort? Adjust your environment and schedule to reduce friction for the ones that were hardest. This iterative approach is how sustainable habits are born.

From My Journey To Yours

I preach about working out. My patients hear it. My family hears it. Anyone who spends more than ten minutes with me probably hears it too. So I want to be honest with you about something: hitting menopause nearly broke my most consistent habit. I was someone who lived in the gym.

Before menopause, before the full weight of business ownership settled in, I was there six days a week—lifting, cycling, moving with intention and joy. Then life did what life does. My husband traveled for extended periods to care for his father. The clinic needed me there for longer hours. My children needed different things from me. Sleep became elusive. Fatigue became constant. And the gym—the thing that had always been my stress release, my clarity, my non-negotiable—got pushed to the back of the line. It happened slowly enough that I almost didn't notice.

And then one day I did notice, and I had to be honest with myself about it.

What eventually worked was not dramatic. It was practical. I stopped expecting myself to maintain the same workout volume I had before menopause and gave myself permission to restructure. Three to four sessions per week instead of six. Walking on the treadmill at home on days I couldn't get to a class. Lifting weights in my basements on evenings when leaving the house wasn't possible. I let go of the guilt and replaced it with gratitude for whatever I could give that day.

I also had to stop being my own biggest obstacle. I had equipment. I had knowledge. I had motivation—buried under exhaustion and overwhelm, but it was there. I just had to reorganize my approach. And when I did, the habit came back— not exactly as it was, but adapted, sustainable, and mine again. That modification was not failure. It was wisdom.

Your Turn To Reflect

Think of a positive habit you have struggled to build or maintain. What made it difficult—and what ultimately helped you either succeed or adapt? How does your experience mirror what the midlife readers of this book are navigating? Write your reflection below.

____

____

____

____

____

CHAPTER 9

Midlife Mind-Body Reset

Motivation, Discipline, and Your Personal Reset

You now have the foundational knowledge: how to fuel your brain through nutrition, how to build strength and mobility through intentional movement, how to manage stress and support recovery, and how to build habits that actually last. The next step is integration—pulling all four pillars together into a structured, actionable program that produces measurable, visible results.

I call this the **Midlife Mind-Body Reset.** It is not a crash course or a 30-day miracle promise. It is a systematic approach to resetting your baseline—physically, neurologically, and mentally—and establishing the daily practices that will carry you forward long after the 30 days have passed.

The Five Steps of the Reset

- **Step 1: Reset Your Nutrition**

Goal: Stabilize energy, reduce inflammation, and fuel your brain and body with intention.

- Eat protein + healthy fat + complex carbohydrate at each meal.

- Include at least one serving of vegetables or fruit per meal.

- Drink 2 liters of water daily—and actually track it.

- Minimize processed foods and refined sugars. Not eliminate—minimize. Progress over perfection.

Practical Tip

*The **'plate method'** is simple and effective: half your plate in vegetables, one quarter in lean protein, one quarter in complex carbohydrates. It requires no calorie counting and no elaborate meal planning.*

- **Step 2: Move With Purpose**

Goal: Rebuild functional strength, stimulate neuroplasticity, and restore mobility.

- Strength training 2–3 sessions per week using exercises from Chapter 6.

- Cardio 20–30 minutes, 2–3 times per week—walking, cycling, HIIT, or any activity you enjoy.

- Mobility practice 5–10 minutes daily, especially before strength sessions.

Practical Tip

Schedule your workouts as calendar appointments the same way you would a medical appointment or a meeting with your most important client. Because this is a meeting with your most important client — yourself.

- **Step 3: Strengthen Your Mindset**

Goal: Build the mental infrastructure that makes all other habits sustainable.

- Five minutes of morning reflection or journaling to set daily intention.

- One to two minutes of visualization—seeing yourself completing your goals with energy and confidence.

- One acknowledged win per day, no matter how small.

- **Step 4: Optimize Recovery**

Goal: Restore the body and brain to perform at their best.

- Aim for 7–9 hours of sleep per night. Consistent sleep and wake times matter.

- Active recovery on rest days: gentle walking, yoga, foam rolling.

- Daily stress management: 5 minutes of deep breathing, meditation, or quiet reflection.

Step 5: Integrate and Sustain

Goal: Make the Reset a lifestyle, not a phase.

- Identify the 3–5 habits that made the biggest difference for you during the Reset.

- Stack those habits onto existing routines for maximum sustainability.

- Track, review, and adjust weekly.

Your 30-Day Reset Timeline

- **Week 1:** Build nutritional awareness and establish morning mindset practice. Focus on food quality and hydration.

- **Week 2:** Add strength training and daily mobility. Begin tracking physical performance.

- **Week 3:** Layer in cardiovascular movement and refine recovery strategies.

- **Week 4:** Integrate all pillars fully. Evaluate progress, celebrate wins, and solidify the habits you're keeping.

From My Journey To Yours

Physical therapy school at Nova Southeastern University was one of the hardest things I have ever done. And I say that as someone who has since run a clinical practice, managed a staff, navigated a family health crisis, and built a business from scratch. NSU was hard in a different way—intellectually, emotionally, and in terms of sheer self-belief.

The program used a problem-based learning model, which meant we were not simply handed lectures and expected to memorize and regurgitate. We were given complex clinical cases and expected to reason through evaluation, diagnosis, and treatment—often without enough information, always under pressure. Most of my classmates hated it. Many of us, including me, had moments of genuine doubt about whether we belonged in that room.

My motivation during those years was not always high. There were days I questioned my path, my preparation, and my capability. What carried me through was not inspiration—it was discipline. And faith. I am a woman of faith, and I genuinely believed that God did not bring me to that program not to bring me through it. That belief was the floor I stood on when motivation failed.

What I have come to understand, looking back, is that the difficulty of that training was not an obstacle—it was the training itself. The problem-based model was building a skill that has defined my entire clinical career: the ability to think. Not to recite protocols, but to analyze, reason, and solve. That capacity has made me one of the strongest clinical thinkers I know—and I say that not with arrogance, but with genuine gratitude for the process that produced it.

The mindset shift that changed everything was this: I stopped seeing the difficulty as evidence of inadequacy and started seeing it as evidence of the quality of what I was building. That reframe— from *'this is too hard'* to *'this is making me excellent'*— is available to anyone. It is what discipline, in its truest form, actually produces.

Your Turn To Reflect

Recall a time when motivation was absent but discipline carried you forward anyway. What mindset shift made the most significant difference? How did pushing through that season shape who you became? Use the space below to reflect on your own experience with discipline and perseverance.

____

____

____

____

____

____

CHAPTER 10

❧

Your 30-Day Action Plan

*Building Sustainable Habits — Your
Blueprint for the Next 30 Days*

Everything we have built together in this book comes down to this: consistent daily action. This chapter is your practical launchpad—a structured, clear, 30-day plan that translates everything you've learned into a daily practice across all four pillars. Use this plan as a framework, not a rigid rulebook. Life will happen. You will miss a day. That is not failure — that is life. What matters is that you return to the plan the next day, without drama and without the kind of perfectionism that kills more health journeys than lack of effort ever will.

Daily Pillar Actions

- **Pillar 1: Nutrition**

1. Eat protein + healthy fat + complex carbohydrate at each meal.

2. At least one serving of vegetables or fruit per meal.

3. Drink 6–8 cups (~2 liters) of water daily.

4. Avoid processed foods and refined sugars as much as possible.

Daily Reflection: What meals energized me today? What would I adjust tomorrow?

Pillar 2: Movement

1. Strength training 2–3 times per week, 20–30 minutes per session.

2. Cardio 2–3 times per week, 20–30 minutes (walking, cycling, or interval work).

3. Mobility and stretching 5–10 minutes daily.

Daily Reflection: What movement felt strong today? What improved — energy, posture, endurance?

Pillar 3: Mindset

1. Morning reflection or journaling: 5 minutes.

2. Visualization: 1–2 minutes, your goals clearly and vividly imagined.

3. Identify and acknowledge one win — no matter how small.

Daily Reflection: What progress did I make today? What obstacle did I navigate?

Pillar 4: Recovery

1. Target 7–9 hours of sleep per night, with consistent sleep and wake times.

2. Active recovery on rest days: gentle movement, yoga, or stretching.

3. 5 minutes of stress management: deep breathing, meditation, or a mindful pause.

Daily Reflection: How did I feel physically and mentally? What recovery strategy helped most?

Weekly Focus

- **Week 1:** Nutrition and mindset foundations. Build awareness, establish habits, track energy.

- **Week 2:** Introduce strength training and daily mobility. Observe physical performance changes.

- **Week 3:** Add cardiovascular movement and refine recovery strategies.

- **Week 4:** Full integration across all four pillars. Evaluate, celebrate, and solidify.

Accountability Practices That Actually Work

- Track daily using a journal or checklist—the act of recording creates awareness and commitment.

- Spend 10–15 minutes every Sunday reviewing the week: wins, challenges, energy trends.

- Celebrate every weekly completion with something meaningful—a massage, new workout gear, time outdoors, a meal you love.

- Find a partner or coach. Shared goals create shared accountability—and make the journey considerably less lonely.

From My Journey To Yours

I'll be transparent about something: being a small business owner has been my greatest life challenge—and my greatest teacher. Most people understand, conceptually, what it means to own a business. Very few understand what it actually feels like to carry one. The weight of payroll, patient care, staff management, clinical documentation, marketing, compliance—and doing it all simultaneously, often without a break.

The habit I struggled most to maintain through the most intense seasons of building my clinic was working out. I say that knowing exactly how ironic it sounds, given that I spend my professional life telling other people to exercise. But that irony is actually the point: even those of us who know better, who preach it with conviction, who have seen the research — we are not immune to life.

At my lowest point of gym consistency, I was making excuses I would never have accepted from a patient. Too tired. Too busy. Too much to do. And underneath those excuses was something deeper: I was carrying guilt for needing rest, and at the same time carrying guilt for not working out. It was an exhausting loop.

The change came when I gave myself permission to modify, not abandon. Three to four days a week instead of six. Twenty minutes instead of an hour when necessary. My home gym instead of the facility when time was tight. I had to let go of the version of myself that worked out at a certain intensity and volume, and meet the version of me that was here right now.

That modification was the habit that saved the habit. And my health. Midlife readers—I want you to hear this: your version of the habit does not have to look like mine, or anyone else's. It has to look like something you can actually sustain. Start there. Refine from there. The direction matters infinitely more than the pace.

Your Turn To Reflect

Think of a positive habit you personally struggled to build or maintain—one that midlife readers will likely recognize in themselves. What made it difficult? What ultimately helped? What would you tell someone who is in the middle of that struggle right now? Write your reflection below.

CHAPTER 11

Case Studies & Success Stories

The Midlife Wellness Reset — Real Transformations,
Real People

Theory is powerful. Research is essential. But when you see real people—people just like you—applying these principles and experiencing genuine transformation, something shifts from the intellectual to the visceral. You begin to believe it's possible not just in theory, but for you. That belief is the bridge between information and action.

The following case studies are composite portraits drawn from the kinds of transformations I witness regularly in my clinical practice and coaching work. They are offered not as promises of identical outcomes, but as evidence that this system works — when applied consistently, with self-compassion and appropriate expectation.

Case Study 1: Sarah, 52 — Reclaiming Energy and Confidence

Sarah was a marketing executive who had spent the better part of a decade putting her career and family ahead of her health. By the time she began the Mind Strong, Body Strong Reset, she was experiencing significant afternoon energy crashes, stubborn weight gain, and a creeping loss of confidence that she couldn't quite name.

She started with small, sustainable changes. A serving of vegetables at every meal. A 20-minute strength session twice a week. Five minutes of morning journaling. Seven to eight hours of sleep. The changes seemed almost too simple to produce meaningful results.

After 30 days, Sarah had lost six pounds—without any dramatic dietary restriction. Her afternoon energy was consistently higher. Her posture had improved. Her back stiffness had reduced noticeably. But what she mentioned most frequently was something harder to measure: she felt like herself again. Sarah's story illustrates what consistent, integrated action across multiple pillars produces: not just physical change, but a restoration of identity and confidence that ripples through every area of life.

Case Study 2: James, 48 — Rebuilding Focus and Mental Stamina

James was a software project manager dealing with significant brain fog, declining physical stamina, and chronic stress that had accumulated over years of high-pressure work. He had tried various health approaches before—individual diet programs, a brief gym phase—but nothing had stuck, because nothing had addressed the full picture.

He began focusing on brain-supportive nutrition—salmon twice a week, daily berries, leafy greens with every meal. He added morning walks and two strength sessions per week. He adopted a brief visualization practice before his workday to set intention. He improved his sleep hygiene by eliminating screens an hour before bed and keeping consistent sleep times.

The result, after 30 days, was not just physical. His cognitive performance at work improved. The afternoon fog lifted. His stress response became less reactive. He described feeling, for the first time in years, like he was ahead of his day rather than behind it. The integration of all four pillars had produced a synergistic effect that no single intervention had managed alone.

Case Study 3: Maria, 55 — Thriving Through Life's Demands

Maria was managing the physical demands of being a primary caregiver while simultaneously dealing with joint stiffness, low energy, and the emotional weight of chronic stress. She had essentially placed her own needs last for so long that she had forgotten what her own good health felt like.

She chose low-impact modifications throughout: gentle strength work to protect her joints, anti-inflammatory nutrition to reduce stiffness, morning reflection to maintain emotional equilibrium, and consistent sleep to rebuild her depleted energy reserves. She also added yoga as both an active recovery practice and a stress-management tool.

Thirty days later, Maria's joint stiffness had reduced meaningfully. Her daily energy was higher and more stable. Her mood had lifted. She described feeling 'more like myself than I have in years'—which, of course, is the goal. Her story demonstrates that the Mind Strong, Body Strong Method is fully adaptable to different fitness levels, life circumstances, and starting points.

What These Stories Share

Consistency is the single most important variable. Even the smallest, most consistent daily actions compound into real and measurable results. Integration amplifies everything. Addressing nutrition, movement, mindset, and recovery simultaneously produces outcomes that no single pillar achieves alone.

Adaptability is a feature, not a compromise. The system works across different bodies, schedules, fitness levels, and life circumstances. Reflection accelerates transformation. Tracking progress and celebrating wins sustains the intrinsic motivation that makes change feel rewarding rather than punishing.

From My Journey To Yours

The topic of this chapter's personal reflection is the reset — and I've spoken in earlier chapters about my personal experience with menopause as a kind of forced reset. But this is where I want to go a layer deeper, into the specific experience of learning to sleep again.

When menopause arrived in earnest, sleep became the most immediate casualty. I had never been someone who struggled with sleep—until suddenly I was. Night waking, hot flashes interrupting deep sleep cycles, the inability to return to sleep after 4 AM. For someone who had always functioned on good sleep and whose clinical performance depended on it, this was disorienting.

My colleague Dr. Katrina Banks, DPT—who co-hosts Neurowellness Conversations with me and has written a book titled "Rest Is Power"—had spoken often about the value of learning to 'wind down.' I had heard her say it many times. It took my own sleep crisis for me to actually implement it. I established a wind-down routine. Consistent bedtime. Cool, dark room with blackout curtains. No screens an hour before bed. No documentation or email in the late evening hours. I had frank conversations with my husband—a devoted night owl—about what the bedroom environment needed to look like. We compromised, as partners do. And the sleep improved.

What followed was a cascade of positive changes: lower cortisol, better focus, more consistent energy, more patience, greater emotional regulation, and a weight-loss response that had been stalled for months. My reset began with sleep—and once that pillar was stabilized, every other pillar responded.

My key message to you is this: investigate what is actually happening in your body, name it clearly, and then build a plan to address it. For me, the reset was sleep. For you, it might be something different. But the process is the same—awareness, intention, and consistent action.

Your Turn To Reflect

Share a personal 'reset' moment—a point when you intentionally changed something significant about your routine, health, or lifestyle. What prompted the reset, what did you change, and what transformation resulted? Use the space below to map your own reset journey.

____

____

____

____

____

____

____

CHAPTER 12

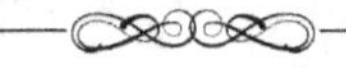

Your Best Life Starts Now

Thriving Forward — This Is Where It Begins

We have arrived at the final chapter together — and I want to acknowledge something: the fact that you have read this far means you are serious. It means you have decided, at some level, that you are worth the investment. And that decision is everything. Reading this book has given you knowledge. Knowledge of how your brain works, how your body responds, and what the science says about nutrition, movement, mindset, and recovery in midlife. That knowledge is real and it is valuable. But it is the beginning of the story, not the end of it.

Transformation happens in the daily practice. It happens in the choice to move when you don't feel like it, to eat intentionally when convenience is calling, to pause and breathe when stress is escalating, and to close the laptop and protect your sleep even when the to-do list says otherwise. Those small, deliberate choices—made consistently, over days and weeks and months — are what change looks like from the inside.

The Four Pillars of Your New Life

- **Nutrition.** Fuel your brain and body with foods that energize, support cognition, and reduce inflammation.

- **Movement.** Strengthen and mobilize your body through consistent, purposeful movement that builds function, not just form.

- **Mindset.** Train your mind to stay motivated, focused, and resilient — even when the season is difficult.

- **Recovery.** Recharge your body and brain with proper sleep, stress management, and intentional recovery.

Your Commitments Going Forward

I want to invite you to make the following commitments — not to me, but to yourself:

I will fuel my body and brain with intention.

I will move my body consistently and purposefully.

I will train my mind to support my goals, not undermine them.

I will prioritize recovery as a strategic tool, not a luxury.

I will build habits that compound — and I will trust the process.

The Power of Momentum

Every choice you make compounds over time. A single healthy meal, a 20-minute walk, a moment of morning reflection, one full night of restorative sleep—none of these things feel dramatic in isolation. But stacked day after day, week after week, month after month, they create extraordinary results. Not the overnight transformation that social media promises, but the deep, durable change that comes from earning it. Your best life is not a destination you arrive at. It is a direction you move in, consistently, with intention and courage.

Go forward. Move with purpose. Nourish your brain. Build your strength. Protect your sleep. Train your mind. And trust that every single step—even the imperfect ones—is carrying you exactly where you are meant to go. Because you deserve nothing less than your best life. And it starts now.

From My Journey To Yours

I have the privilege of being trusted by some of the most courageous people I have ever met. They walk—and sometimes are wheeled—through my clinic doors carrying diagnoses that would make many of us fold. And instead, they show up, session after session, choosing to fight for their own function and their own lives.

One patient stands out as the embodiment of thriving forward. I'll call him Zion. He was a music producer—young, successful, full of creative energy—who had built a life around his work. Like so many of us who are building something we love, Zion had ignored the signals his body was sending. His blood pressure had been elevated for a while. He knew it. He didn't address it. And one day, he had a stroke. He was under 55. He was vibrant and had a full life ahead of him. And in one moment, that life required a complete pivot.

When Zion found his way to my clinic, he had heard we were among the best in the region for neurological rehabilitation. He came with two things that are the rarest and most valuable combination I see in a patient: humility to accept help, and relentless work ethic. I told him the work would be hard. He didn't blink. I built the most comprehensive plan I could for his recovery. He brought everything he had to every single session. He thrived. Genuinely. When he left my care, he had minimal to no residual signs of his stroke. He returned to his career, to his life, to his purpose. He took what looked like an ending and made it a turning point.

Zion's story is the story I carry with me into every difficult season of my own. My father used to preach about taking lemons and making lemonade. Life will always provide the lemons. What we choose to do with them—whether we make something with them or let them sit and rot—that is entirely within our power. Zion chose lemonade. I've tried to do the same every day since. And I hope, after reading this book, that you will too.

Your Turn To Reflect

Offer your own story about a time when you—or someone you admire—embraced a new direction with courage. What did that look like? What did thriving forward mean in that season? And what does thriving forward mean to you right now? Use the space below to write the next chapter of your own story.

____

____

____

____

____

____

____

MIND STRONG, BODY STRONG

COMPANION TOOLKIT

Your Daily Tools for Transformation

Tool 1: 30-Day Daily Habit Tracker

Day	Nutrition ✔	Movement ✔	Mindset ✔	Recovery ✔	Notes & Reflections
1					
2					
3					
4					
5					
6					
7					
8					
9					
10					

Day	Nutrition ✔	Movement ✔	Mindset ✔	Recovery ✔	Notes & Reflections
11					
12					
13					
14					
15					
16					
17					
18					
19					
20					

Day	Nutrition ✔	Movement ✔	Mindset ✔	Recovery ✔	Notes & Reflections
21					
22					
23					
24					
25					
26					
27					
28					
29					
30					

Use this tracker every day to monitor your consistency across all four pillars. Place a checkmark (✔) in each column that applies. Use the Notes column to track energy levels, mood shifts, physical changes, or insights. Reviewing this at the end of each week is one of the most powerful practices in this program.

Tool 2: Weekly Reflection Worksheet

Complete this at the end of each week. The practice of reviewing your week — wins, challenges, and patterns — builds the self-awareness that sustains long-term change.

- **Week 1**

Wins & Progress — What did I accomplish this week?

____

____

____

____

Challenges — What obstacles did I face? How did I respond?

____

____

____

Energy & Mood — How did I feel physically and mentally?

____

____

____

Adjustments for Next Week — What will I change or improve?

____

____

____

____

• **Week 2**

Wins & Progress — What did I accomplish this week?

____

____

____

____

Challenges — What obstacles did I face? How did I respond?

____

____

____

____

Energy & Mood — How did I feel physically and mentally?

____

____

____

Adjustments for Next Week — What will I change or improve?

____

____

- **Week 3**

Wins & Progress — What did I accomplish this week?

____

____

____

Challenges — What obstacles did I face? How did I respond?

____

____

Energy & Mood — How did I feel physically and mentally?

____

____

Adjustments for Next Week — What will I change or improve?

____

____

____

- **Week 4**

Wins & Progress — What did I accomplish this week?

____

____

____

____

Challenges — What obstacles did I face? How did I respond?

____

____

____

____

Energy & Mood — How did I feel physically and mentally?

____

____

____

Adjustments for Next Week — What will I change or improve?

____

____

____

____

Tool 3: 7-Day Nutrition Log

Track every meal, snack, and hydration intake for one week. The goal is not restriction or calorie counting — it is awareness. What you track, you can improve.

Day	Meals	Snacks	Hydration	Notes (Energy, Cravings, Mood)
Monday				
Tuesday				
Wednesday				
Thursday				
Friday				
Saturday				
Sunday				

Tool 4: 30-Day Movement & Mobility Log

Use this log to record your physical activity across all three movement categories: strength, cardio, and mobility. Note your energy and performance observations in the final column. Seeing your activity record grow week by week is one of the most motivating tools you have.

Day	Strength Exercises	Cardio ✔	Mobility / Stretch ✔	Notes (Energy, Performance)
Day 1				
Day 2				
Day 3				
Day 4				
Day 5				
Day 6				
Day 7				
Day 8				

Day	Strength Exercises	Cardio ✔	Mobility / Stretch ✔	Notes (Energy, Performance)
Day 9				
Day 10				
Day 11				
Day 12				
Day 13				
Day 14				
Day 15				
Day 16				

Day	Strength Exercises	Cardio ✔	Mobility / Stretch ✔	Notes (Energy, Performance)
Day 17				
Day 18				
Day 19				
Day 20				
Day 21				
Day 22				
Day 23				
Day 24				

Day	Strength Exercises	Cardio ✔	Mobility / Stretch ✔	Notes (Energy, Performance)
Day 25				
Day 26				
Day 27				
Day 28				
Day 29				
Day 30				

Tool 5: Daily Mindset & Journaling Practice

These four reflection prompts are designed to build the self-awareness and positive reinforcement loops that sustain motivation and behavioral change. Use them every morning or evening — or both. Five minutes of intentional reflection each day will compound into profound self-knowledge over 30 days.

1. What am I genuinely grateful for today?

____

____

____

____

2. What small win did I accomplish — and did I acknowledge it?

____

____

____

____

3. How did I challenge myself or move closer to my goals today?

____

____

____

____

4. What is the one thing I will focus on tomorrow to maintain momentum?

____

____

____

____

____

Visualization Practice

- Once daily—morning or evening— close your eyes for 1–2 minutes.

- Picture yourself completing your daily goals with energy, confidence, and ease.

- See the details: what you're wearing, where you are, how your body feels.

- Feel the satisfaction of having done the work.

- Open your eyes and write one intention for the day below:

My intention for today:

____

____

____

____

____

Tool 6: 30-Day Challenge Calendar

Use this visual calendar to check off each completed day. Mark the pillars you completed with their initials: N (Nutrition), M (Movement), Mi (Mindset), R (Recovery). A complete day earns all four. Visual momentum is a powerful motivator — watch your calendar fill up.

MON	TUE	WED	THU	FRI	SAT	SUN
Day 1	Day 2	Day 3	Day 4	Day 5	Day 6	Day 7
Day 8	Day 9	Day 10	Day 11	Day 12	Day 13	Day 14
Day 15	Day 16	Day 17	Day 18	Day 19	Day 20	Day 21
Day 22	Day 23	Day 24	Day 25	Day 26	Day 27	Day 28
Day 29	Day 30					

Tool 7: Mind Strong, Body Strong Quick Reference Guide

Keep this summary close as a daily reminder of your foundational practices across all four pillars.

NUTRITION — Fuel Your Brain & Body

- Eat protein + healthy fat + complex carb at every meal

- Include vegetables or fruit at every meal

- Drink 2 liters of water daily — track it

- Prioritize anti-inflammatory foods: fatty fish, berries, leafy greens, nuts.

- Limit processed foods and refined sugars

- Eat every 3–4 hours to stabilize blood sugar and energy

MOVEMENT — Strengthen and Mobilize

- Strength training 2–3 times per week, 20–30 minutes

- Cardiovascular movement 2–3 times per week, 20–30 minutes

- Daily mobility and stretching, 5–10 minutes minimum

- Start with bodyweight if equipment is unavailable

- Focus on form before intensity — always

- Choose activities you enjoy to sustain consistency

MINDSET — Train Your Mind

- 5 minutes of morning reflection or journaling daily

- 1–2 minutes of daily visualization — see yourself succeeding

- Celebrate one win per day, no matter how small

- Reframe setbacks as information, not failure

- Find an accountability partner or community

- Review your goals every 3–6 months

RECOVERY — Recharge and Restore

- Target 7–9 hours of sleep per night with consistent timing

- Limit screens 60 minutes before bedtime

- Include active recovery on rest days — walking, yoga, stretching

- Practice 5 minutes of deep breathing or meditation daily

- Track energy levels to identify your best recovery strategies

- Protect your sleep environment: cool, dark, and quiet.

Connect With Dr. Paulette

Continue Your Journey

This book is the beginning of a conversation—not the end of one. If the stories, strategies, and science in these pages have resonated with you, I want you to know that there is more available to you.

Join the Community

I have built communities where real people apply the Mind Strong, Body Strong principles together—sharing wins, navigating challenges, and holding each other accountable. I would love to welcome you.

- **Online Community:** Search 'Mind Strong Body Strong' on your preferred platform

- **Parkinson's Boxing Program:** Contact the clinic directly for program information

- **Neurowellness Conversations Podcast:** Co-hosted with Dr. Katrina Banks, DPT

Work With Me Directly

For those who want personalized guidance—whether for general health and wellness coaching, neurological physical therapy consultation, or support navigating the specific challenges of midlife—I am available for one-on-one work.

- Health & Wellness Coaching and Consultation

- Neurological Physical Therapy Services

- Corporate Wellness Education and Speaking Engagements

Reach out through my clinic or website to begin a conversation about what support would serve you best.

You deserve nothing less than your best life.

Go forward. Thrive.

— *Dr. Paulette Lewis, DPT*

MIND STRONG, BODY STRONG

References & Bibliography

Dr. Paulette Lewis, DPT | Doctor of Neurological Physical Therapy

A Note on This Reference Section

This bibliography presents, in APA 7th Edition format, all peer-reviewed research studies and scientific sources cited within Mind Strong, Body Strong. The references are organized alphabetically by first author's surname.

Each entry is followed by a note indicating which chapter(s) of the book cite that source, to assist readers who wish to locate and explore the original research. Where a DOI (Digital Object Identifier) is available, it is provided for direct digital access to the source.

Note to readers: Several claims in this book are supported by well-established scientific consensus (e.g., the brain-body connection, neuroplasticity, benefits of exercise for cognitive function) that are grounded in the foundational neuroscience literature rather than a single citable study. The references below represent the specific studies that are cited directly in the text.

References

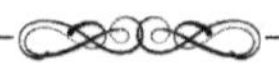

R

Raichle, M. E., & Gusnard, D. A. (2002). Appraising the brain's energy budget. Proceedings of the National Academy of Sciences of the United States of America, 99(16), 10237–10239. https://doi.org/10.1073/pnas.172399499

S

Salvy, S.-J., Roemmich, J. N., Bowker, J. C., Romero, N. D., Stadler, P. J., & Epstein, L. H. (2009). Effect of peers and friends on youth physical activity and motivation to be physically active. Journal of Pediatric Psychology, 34(2), 217–225. https://doi.org/10.1093/jpepsy/jsn071

Sartori, A. C., Vance, D. E., Slater, L. Z., & Crowe, M. (2012). The impact of inflammation on cognitive function in older adults: Implications for healthcare practice and research. Journal of Neuroscience Nursing, 44(4), 206–217. https://doi.org/10.1097/JNN.0b013e3182527690

Additional Foundational Sources

The following sources represent the scientific literature that informs the foundational principles of the Mind Strong, Body Strong Method — including the neuroscience of neuroplasticity, the role of exercise in brain health, and the evidence base for nutrition in cognitive function. These works are not individually cited in the text but constitute the evidence base underlying the book's core framework. They are provided here for readers who wish to explore the primary research literature.

C

Cotman, C. W., & Berchtold, N. C. (2002). Exercise: A behavioral intervention to enhance brain health and plasticity. Trends in Neurosciences, 25(6), 295–301. https://doi.org/10.1016/S0166-2236(02)02143-4

Erickson, K. I., Voss, M. W., Prakash, R. S., Basak, C., Szabo, A., Chaddock, L., Kim, J. S., Heo, S., Alves, H., White, S. M., Wojcicki, T. R., Mailey, E., Vieira, V. J., Martin, S. A., Pence, B. D., Woods, J. A., McAuley, E., & Kramer, A. F. (2011). Exercise training increases size of hippocampus and improves memory. Proceedings of the National Academy of Sciences of the United States of America, 108(7), 3017–3022. https://doi.org/10.1073/pnas.1015 950108

M

Morris, M. C., Evans, D. A., Tangney, C. C., Bienias, J. L., & Wilson, R. S. (2006). Associations of vegetable and fruit consumption with age-related cognitive change. Neurology, 67(8), 1370–1376. https://doi.org/10.1212/01.wnl.0000240224.38978.d8

P

Ploughman, M. (2008). Exercise is brain food: The effects of physical activity on cognitive function. Developmental Neurorehabilitation, 11(3), 236–240. https://doi.org/10.1080/17518420801997007

S

Sofi, F., Abbate, R., Gensini, G. F., & Casini, A. (2010). Accruing evidence on benefits of adherence to the Mediterranean diet on health: An updated systematic review and meta-analysis. The American Journal of Clinical Nutrition, 92(5), 1189–1196. https://doi.org/10.3945/ajcn.2010.29673

W

Walker, M. P. (2017). Why we sleep: Unlocking the power of sleep and dreams. Scribner.

Online & Non-Journal Sources Cited

J

Jamadar, S. (2023, January 25). How much energy do we expend thinking and using our brain? The Conversation. https://doi.org/10.64628/AA.emxrxg7sf

Author's Note on Citations and Future Editions

As a clinician and researcher, I am committed to grounding the content of this book in peer-reviewed science. In future editions of Mind Strong, Body Strong, I intend to expand the reference section to include in-text citation numbers corresponding to each specific claim.

Readers who wish to explore the research base further are encouraged to visit PubMed (pubmed.ncbi.nlm.nih.gov) and Google Scholar (scholar.google.com), where all peer-reviewed sources referenced in this bibliography are freely accessible or available through most public library systems.

For questions regarding the scientific basis of any claim in this book, please reach out through my clinic or website. I welcome the conversation.

— Dr. Paulette Lewis, DPT

About The Author

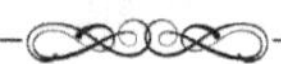

Dr. Paulette Lewis, MPT, DPT is a doctor of neurological physical therapy, a certified stroke rehabilitation specialist, and a certified Parkinson's therapist who has been a clinician and educator for over 26 years. Dr. Lewis additionally holds certifications in LDBF Parkinson's Boxing, through the Center of Movement Challenges out of Atlanta, Georgia, a Certification as a Stroke Rehabilitation Specialist, and in Dry Needling and Ultrasound Dry Needling. She has been a clinic owner for over nine years. Her clinic is one of two neurological out-patient therapy practices in the South Metro Atlanta area. What sets her clinic apart, however, is the specialized training that she and her staff have with regard to neurological patients. Dr. Lewis' clinic provides top-notch innovative treatments that are all based on current research. Proudly, she is a devoted wife, mother of two beautiful children, and the daughter of two retired teachers and ministers of the gospel.

Dr. Lewis wrote this book with her patients, her friends, and their friends, in mind. The transition into mid-life dealt her some challenges that she had to find the answer to, in order to get her health and her life back. Those tools discovered made the difference, and she realized that if she was struggling through it, others had to be as well. And yes, communications with friends, and friends of friends, proved just that. She realized that she needed to share this information, and began to put pen to paper to do just that. That resulted in this book and journal, which she so appropriately titled, ***"Mind Strong, Body Strong."***

Once you've read this book you will be equipped with the tools necessary to move into your best health. You will have the steps to make your health better, both physically and mentally. Join Dr. Lewis though her YouTube community, and social media pages, to share your journey. Additionally, if you need further guidance to improve your health and wellness, or you need help in ensuring that your rehabilitation plan is what's best for you, then you can reach out to Dr. Lewis through her website for a consultation. Now, your call to action is to move your body, put real foods in your body, challenge your mind and rest your body.

9 798999 611560